PURE FAT BURNING FOOD

The Easy, Healthy Way To Permanent Fat Loss With ZERO Calorie Counting!

by Jennifer James

Published in Great Britain by:

LeadsClick
26 York Street
London
W1U 6PZ

© Copyright 2013 – Jennifer James

ISBN-13: 978-1494372415
ISBN-10: 149437241X

Table of Contents

INTRODUCTION: WHY YOU SHOULD IGNORE THE WEIGHT LOSS & FOOD INDUSTRY

Take a look around and you are bound to notice there is a problem which is spreading quickly and beginning to affect more and more of those around us.

...It may even be starting to affect **you and your family.**

This burgeoning problem is a propensity towards weight gain. The number of overweight and obese people in the world is on the rise. With the ease and convenience of fast food and busy lifestyles, which prevent many of us from exercising regularly, weight gain seems almost inevitable.

However, you don't have to be overweight or obese.

While the number of obese individuals seems to rise on a daily basis, it also seems as though each passing day sees the introduction of a new miracle diet pill, fad diet or cleverly labeled foods aimed at eliminating the problem.

However, despite the increasing number of diet products

on the market the obesity epidemic continues to fester. The unfortunate reason for this is these pills and products marketed as miracle solutions are not only poor excuses for diet aids, but they may even be compounding the obesity problem.

In this report we will examine how the weight loss and food industry is profiting while doing nothing to help solve the problem of obesity. We will also highlight the food groups that are proven to help shed fat quickly and those you should avoid as much as possible.

The information contained in this report may not be ground breaking or revolutionary but it will be beneficial to readers who are legitimately trying to lose weight the right and most effective way.

Fad diets may come and go and the weight loss industry seems to introduce new pills and supplements for the purpose of helping lose weight but these diet aids simply do not work.

In reading this report you will understand how consumers have become pawns in the industry simply because so few people understand how proper nutrition and exercise can help them enjoy both trimmer waistlines and better overall health.

Weight Loss Industry Profits While Consumers Suffer

Obesity is becoming an increasingly prevalent problem and as a result the weight loss industry is booming. However, despite an increase in the number of drugs available and fad diets being introduced, as a nation we are not losing weight.

How can this be?

It would seem if new drugs and diets are being introduced each year, the number of obese citizens would be on the decline as more and more members of society turn to these pills and diets in an effort to lose weight.

However, this logic is flawed because of one basic fact...

The vast majority of these drugs and fad diets do not work.

In fact they may only be serving to exacerbate the problem of obesity by providing consumers with a false sense of hope that these pills or fad diets will help them to lose weight and achieve optimal health.

Unsuspecting consumers watch commercials or read advertisements with claims of substantial weight loss simply by using a product or following a fad diet.

These advertisements touting excellent weight loss results with minimal effort seem too good to be true. Consumers get caught up in believing these products will provide them with the answer to their weight problem but the truth of the matter is...

...weight loss does not come in a bottle.

However, when consumers are duped by these advertisements they continue to pump money into the ever-growing weight loss industry. Some estimates place the amount of money Americans spend on weight loss products and services at roughly $33 billion per year.

With so much money invested in this industry each year in conjunction with obesity rates which continue to rise, it is clear consumers are being deceived and while those in the weight loss industry continue to profit, our waistlines continue to expand and our wallets continue to shrink.

So, how do consumers know if a weight loss product is worth the investment?

The answer to this seemingly complex question is actually rather quite simple. The most sound piece of advice we can offer to those seeking a way to lose weight is to assume solutions which seem too good to be true, should be avoided.

Instead of relying on miracle weight loss situations it is more important to focus on a more realistic approach to weight loss. You probably are already well aware that proper nutrition and exercise are necessary for effective weight loss.

Therefore you can easily determine any weight loss pills, potions or products claiming you do not have to diet or exercise to lose weight **should not be believed.**

Once consumers become more informed, hopefully they begin to realize the vast majority of the diet industry is designed to fatten the wallets of those promoting pills, potions, products and fad diets and NOT to trim the waistlines of those investing in these products.

Anyway ... enough about that, let's focus on YOU, and what you can do to burn fat and live a healthier lifestyle.

Because an even more worrying trend is that towards our food and how it is now produced with bulking agents, cheap fillers and substitutes which make fat loss a nightmare for those unaware of the situation.

And that, is what this report is about ...

Why You Will Never Need Another Weight Loss Plan!

I'm going to take a wild guess ...

This is not the only report you've read on losing weight right?

And the fact that you're here reading this, means you were not successful in losing or keeping the weight off and you're looking for another solution.

Don't be discouraged.

The simple fact is, most fad diets will NEVER work and in the next chapter, I'll explain why.

But, I want you to make a commitment, not just to me, but to yourself.

Read this report with an open mind, and PLEASE, put into action what I reveal to you. I want to get you off the diet treadmill once and for all, end the confusion and put you onto the road of a healthy lifestyle.

Years of trial and error (on myself) and research of the best nutritionists in the world have gone into this report, and IT WORKS!

I can't promise you you'll lose weight rapidly, everyone's lifestyle is different and unless I can be there with you 24 hours a day for the next 14 days, I can't guarantee you those results.

That's up to you.

But, I guarantee this ... If you put into action what you learn here, you'll NEVER look back. You'll burn fat, have more energy, feel more positive, and unlike conventional diets, you'll lose weight and keep it off!

Now I want you to make me a promise, ok?

Follow this for the next 14 days and measure your results ... if you don't feel I've delivered a solid nutritional plan that you can follow that burns fat consistently, I want you to get a refund.

I'm serious. There is so much mis-information in the diet industry and this report is not intended to add to the confusion, but give you nutritionally sound eating plan you can follow with stellar results.

If you feel I've failed on that promise, I don't deserve your money.

The Problem With Diets & Why They Will NEVER Work

Conventional wisdom says to cut calories and exercise more.

This is WRONG as people believe that they can just eat less of the junk they are already eating, exercise, and they will magically start losing weight.

While it's true that taking in less calories than you burn off everyday will lead to a reduction in weight, that's not the whole story and it's far from an effective way to lose weight.

You may lose weight initially, but you will NEVER keep it off.

What in fact happens when you cut calories from your diet, is that your body detects the reduction in calories, and starts going into starvation mode.

This is a survival instinct of your body that will slow down your metabolism so that your body starts burning LESS calories.

It's a vicious circle that reduces your body's natural ability to burn fat. Even when you're sleeping your body is burning fat, but slow down your metabolism with a reduction in calories, and you'll never lose weight permanently, you'll just leave yourself nutrient deprived, constantly hungry and totally miserable because the food cravings will drive you crazy.

Typical diets, also do not account for nutrient density, processing of foods, cheap bulking agents and the effects these have on your hormones.

If all you're eating is empty calories with no nutritious value, you're destined for life on the "diet treadmill" with NO end in sight. The 'secret' is to focus on the nutrient density of the food you're consuming.

Another problem with diets is the word itself ... 'Diet' ... which conditions us to believe that we need to restrict food in order to lose weight.

That is not the case. Your body is a remarkable machine, and eating when you are hungry and finishing when you are full is the right way to eat. Ironically!

As long as your food choices are nutritious and healthy you're on the right track. If all you are eating is highly nutrient food, your body will not crave junk, and this, makes calorie counting redundant.

Counting calories just adds to the confusion, and is not necessary.

Once you learn how to eat the RIGHT foods and AVOID the bad foods, you'll notice a huge change in your body, your mind and your metabolism.

And because you're eating nutritious foods, your cravings

will subside.

With the abundance of diets on the market It's no wonder the majority of people are confused about what it takes to lose weight and stay healthy.

Inside this report, I hope to alleviate that confusion by giving you a detailed plan of foods you should avoid and the foods you should be eating to burn fat and achieve optimum health and wellbeing.

Why You're Overweight & What You Can Do About It

The reason you're overweight is because of the overconsumption of foods that are rich is starchy carbs, refined flours, refined sugar, trans fats AND other genetically modified or processed junk that has no nutritional value and your body cannot use.

Your body is a remarkably efficient machine, but like your car, it needs the correct fuel to function correctly.

Over the last fifty years or so, the food industry (in search of ever increasing profits) has introduced far too many genetically modified and convenience foods into our modern diets.

These foods are loaded with chemicals, additives and preservatives (including high amounts of salt and sugar) that are not supposed to be there. Chronic overconsumption of these foods causes the breakdown of metabolism in two major ways. First, the liver, which is responsible for removing toxic substances from our bodies, is overworked.

When the liver cannot keep up, excess toxins are stored in fat cells.

In addition, another important role that the liver is meant to play - a role in the metabolism of fat, protein and carbohydrates - is neglected because the liver is too busy trying to clear toxins out of the body. In short, when you eat foods that are loaded with junk, your metabolism slows down and you gain weight.

In order to lose weight you need to cut down on the bad calories from your diet.

As time goes on, losing weight becomes harder and harder. That's because poor diets also affect the release of insulin by your pancreas. The pancreas begins to release far more insulin that it should in an effort to control blood sugar spikes that result directly from eating too many refined foods.

Over time, you become resistant to the amount of insulin that is being released and your body releases even more. This overproduction of insulin causes weight gain. It is also a major risk factor for Type II diabetes. If you continue your poor eating habit's, the whole system will eventually shut down.

But It's NOT your fault ... well not entirely.

The problem is, we've brainwashed into believing conventional wisdom from the profit focused food industry, which in many cases are not required to ensure our food is fit for consumption - that's the job of our food governing bodies, which often look in the other direction when warned about 'possible' health risks from expert scientists.

I'm taking about 'cheap' bulking agents, genetically

modified "laboratory created" foods and fillers that are ever present in foods on today's supermarket shelves.

Your body was not created to eat junk like that.

Anyway, I want you to read the following chapters with an open mind, and then go on to research further (if you want to) to further solidify what I am telling you.

If you want to lose weight, it's more important to pay attention to what you eat, rather than how much!

You're constantly hungry, because the majority of your diet comes from genetically modified and carbohydrate rich foods, most of which contain refined sugars, which have an effect on your hormones and your metabolism and make you store fat.

When you consume carbohydrate rich or highly processed foods, depending on the Glycemic Index of that food you get a rush of sugar into your bloodstream, the higher on the GI scale, the more sugar will flood your system.

In order to remove this sugar from your blood and turn it into glucose that your body can use as fuel, your body releases a hormone called 'insulin' to transfer the glucose into the liver.

If you consume too many refined foods and your energy stores are already full, the excess gets stored as ... yep, you guessed it, FAT!

So in order to control the insulin release, we need to have a more stable blood sugar level, and that requires you to eat foods that don't contain refined flours, sugars or highly processed empty calories.

The problem is ... they are EVERYWHERE!

However, there is hope and with smart food choices, you can lose weight, have more energy, and live a healthier lifestyle ... while still enjoying the odd treat.

You've no doubt heard the phrase, ... "you are what you eat".

Well think about this for second...

Did you know that your stomach lining is regenerated every 7-14 days?

Did you also know that you will have a new layer of skin by next month?

And did you know that EVERY cell in your body, yup ... EVERY single one of the 75 trillion cells in your body will be a brand NEW cell within the next 300 days?

That's right, every cell in your body is constantly being broken down and regenerated, and that is fuelled by the foods we eat.

95% of the way we look, feel, behave and operate is determined by our diet.

Did you get that?

Just read that sentence again and take it to heart...

Done? ok ... Are you ready for a new, healthier, leaner YOU?

You are? Good, let's begin.

THE FOODS TO AVOID THAT EVEN YOUR DOCTOR WILL NEVER TELL YOU ABOUT!

Refined Flours & Grains

Conventional wisdom has long advocated for a diet high in grains. As a result grains and refined flours are everywhere; found in nearly every packaged food on the shelf. Though often inexpensive, versatile, tasty, and even addictive, refined flours and grains are major offenders in the quest for weight loss.

Why they're harmful: Most people inherently know that a diet that includes frequent consumption of pastries, cakes, and cookies will certainly result in weight gain.

However, many are surprised to find that it is not just the sugar that poses the problem. Processed grains and refined flours play havoc with the body's insulin response system causing high blood sugar levels leading to weight gain, inflammation, heart disease, and Type II diabetes.

Foods containing them also block the body's ability to absorb and utilize essential vitamins, minerals, and antioxidants.

Where you find them: Refined flours are present in

nearly all bakery goods, breads, cookies, and pre-packaged sweets. Conventional pastas and crackers (even healthy ones) are also made from high levels of refined flours. Breakfast cereals, even those claiming to be healthy, are fully-grain-based and usually contain refined flours, not to mention sweeteners.

Negative impact on weight loss: When refined flours and low-quality grains are ingested, the body undergoes an insulin response that prompts the body to store fat. Inflammation drags down the metabolism and saps the energy you need for exercise and healthy activity.

These foods also spur intense cravings, causing over-consumption of food; especially sweet, salty, fatty, unhealthy foods.

Don't be fooled: Enriched flour is not a healthy substitute. Whole grain and all-natural are also misleading terms as wheat in any form can still cause the heightened insulin response, inflammation, and cravings that halt any effort at weight loss. Products containing corn can also be detrimental to weight loss and cause inflammation.

How to get rid of them: While gluten-free options exist, when it comes to weight loss, there is no substitute for a simple elimination of processed, pre-packaged, grain-based foods. If you must have bread, seek sprouted, whole grain, gluten free options. Within a few days of total elimination, cravings will subside.

Positive impact of elimination: Many people who have long consumed processed grain and refined flour products are shocked at how much better they feel without them. That gassy, bloated feeling that many assumed was just a natural part of eating, is gone. Puffiness subsides, mental clarity increases, energy returns, and the pounds start to melt off.

High Fructose Corn Syrup

High fructose corn syrup, a chemical, laboratory-produced derivative of sugar is hidden in a staggering number of the processed and pre-packaged foods found in a conventional grocery store.

Though commercial food companies claim the safety and natural quality of this chemical, it is unquestionably one of the main causes of obesity and obesity-related illnesses in developed countries.

Where you find it: High fructose corn syrup is commonly found in condiments, frozen meals, breakfast cereals, low-calorie and lite crackers, cookies, and baked goods, pre-packaged desserts, candy, granola bars, alcoholic drink mixes, soda and other flavoured beverages, and sports drinks.

Why It's harmful: High fructose corn syrup causes a spike in blood sugar levels and insulin production. The body, not designed to ingest such a highly chemical product, struggles to digest it.

Obesity-related health conditions, diabetes, and heart disease are the natural outcome of a diet that includes high fructose corn syrup. As the product is typically produced from genetically modified corn, it is impossible to fully estimate the long-term side effects.

Negative impact on weight loss: While sugar is

never advocated as part of a healthy weight loss plan, high fructose corn syrup is an even greater offender as it is so readily converted to fat in the body. The consumption of foods containing high fructose corn syrup naturally means lesser consumption of the nutrient rich foods the body requires for proper functioning and weight loss.

Foods high in high fructose corn syrup also fail to provide natural feelings of satiety that help to discourage excess eating. As a result, a disproportionate number of empty calories are consumed while natural, healthy foods are neglected.

How to get rid of it: Eliminating high fructose corn syrup requires concentrated, savvy label reading. Remember, products that lack packaging also lack this harmful chemical so the more whole, unprocessed foods you consume, the less room in your diet for artificial, weight-loss inhibiting substances.

Switch out soda and sweetened fruit beverages for water or naturally brewed teas. Shop the perimeter of the store for whole foods and skip the processed, packaged, chemically sweetened stuff in the centre aisles.

Positive impact of elimination: Eliminating high fructose corn syrup will retrain your taste buds to what sweet should actually taste like. As you begin to appreciate the natural flavours of whole foods, you will experience diminished cravings for chemical, processed foods. Your body also gets a break from the non-stop sugar spike and insulin response, allowing it to work on burning that fat!

Fake Fats & Refined Oils

Though conventional diet wisdom advocates for the elimination of animal fats and natural oils, it is the chemically processed fats and cheaply made refined vegetable oils that present the genuine threat to weight loss and maintenance of good health.

Where you find them: Chemically processed fats and refined oils are packaged under the following names: partially or fully hydrogenated vegetable oil, corn oil, canola oil, sunflower oil, soybean oil, margarine, Oleo, butter substitutes, and Crisco.

These harmful fats are found in fried foods, processed, pre-packaged snacks, cookies, and desserts, TV dinners, whipped toppings, French fries and other fast food menu items, store-bought cake icing, processedcheese, and dairy substitutes such as coffee creamer.

Why theyre harmful: In these oils the ratio of Omega-6 to Omega-3 fatty acids is disproportionately skewed in favour of the Omega-6s, causing a host of negative physiological chemical reactions.

Overconsumption of these fats is linked to inflammation, autoimmune conditions, blood clots, cancer, and cardiovascular disease. They are especially toxic when heated and reheated under extreme heats.

Negative impact on weight loss: These chemicals

have the power to alter cell walls within the body and to inhibit normal metabolic ability. Result: resistance to weight loss. These fats also fail to provide the satiety that is a side benefit of natural fats and oils. The result is hunger, overconsumption, and inability to lose weight.

How to get rid of them: Look at how your food is prepared. Are you making it home in your kitchen with whole ingredients or are you picking up fast food or warming a frozen dinner in the microwave? Eliminating fake fats and refined oils begins with examining the labels of the foods you are purchasing and committing to preparing whole, natural foods.

Clean the vegetable oil, canola oil, margarine etc. out of the cabinet and refrigerator and replace with coconut oil and olive oil for cooking. Make your own salad dressings and desserts using natural ingredients. Avoid all fried foods.

Positive impact of elimination: Switching out fake, refined fats for organic, natural fats such as butter, olive oil, nuts, seeds, and avocado aids your body's natural metabolic processes, improves the taste of your foods, helps you to feel full and satisfied after meals, and keeps you from feeling hungry in between meals. When the body is accustomed to satiety, it will more naturally and readily release excess weight.

Artificial Sweeteners

Think that diet sodas and calorie-free sweeteners are the ticket to weight loss? Think again. Though often marketed as a weight-conscious option, artificial sweeteners are anything but.

Like high fructose corn syrup, artificial sweeteners are laboratory-created products that inhibit weight loss and have no place in a healthy weight loss program.

Where you find them: The following are artificial, chemically concocted sweeteners: aspartame (aka NutraSweet), Sucralose (aka Splenda), saccharin (aka Sweet 'N' Low), and acesulfame potassium (aka Ace-K, Sunett, Sweet One) and Neotame.

You'll find them in diet sodas and other calorie-free drinks, sugar-free gums, candies, syrups, and jams, as well as any other processed food or dessert product labelled sugar-free or diet.

Why theyre harmful: Artificial sweeteners can be up to 100 times as sweet as sugar causing the individual to constantly crave sweeter and sweeter foods. They are toxic in the body and studies have identified various chemical sweeteners as cancer causing.

Many consumers of artificial sweeteners also report symptoms typical of allergic reactions, as well as headaches, nausea, and a long list of abnormal reactions including psychological side effects as well.

Negative impact on weight loss: These products are chemicals and thus cause chemical reactions within the body, the least of which involves stimulation of the appetite and the suppression of feelings of satiety; a bad combination for weight loss. Studies have also shown that people consuming diet soda with a meal eat significan'tly more than those who consume water or nothing at all.

Some sweeteners also suppress the area of the brain that controls cravings. And although these products contain no real sugar, they nonetheless have the power to fool the body, trigger an insulin response, and cause the body to store calories as fat.

How to get rid of them: With toxins such as these, there is no middle ground. They must be eliminated completely. Going sugar-free doesnt mean replacing sugar with harmful chemicals, it means cutting sugar and It's mutations out of the diet completely.

Start by eliminating soda and calorie-free sweetened beverages with naturally flavoured sparkling water. Clean your cupboards of any product labelled diet. If a sweet flavour is required, use natural sweeteners such as organic honey, maple syrup, or stevia.

Positive impact of elimination: It is hard to estimate the benefits of removing these toxins until they are actually eliminated as they cause different reactions in each individual. In addition to decreased cravings and balanced insulin response, elimination of artificial sweeteners may also bring physiological and psychological benefits.

Commercially Raised Meats & Farmed Fish

Where you find them: The butchers counter or seafood section of your standard supermarket is stocked with commercially raised corn fed beef and farm raised fish. If the label does not specifically indicate that the beef or meat has been grass fed or that the fish is wild caught, you can assume it has been raised using methods that are both inhumane and unnatural for the animal, and unhealthy for you.

Why theyre harmful: Just like the packaged and processed foods that are so detrimental to your health and counterproductive to your weight loss goals, commercially raised meats and fishes are also factory foods. The methods that farmers and fisheries use to increase the weight and number of these animals are not neutral procedures; they affect the health and chemical composition of the finished product and ultimately the health of you.

Not only are these sources of protein then lower in nutrient value, they also contain byproducts such as hormones, antibiotics, higher levels of omega-6s, and a higher level of acidity. E.coli is also more prevalent among grain fed, feedlot animals.

Negative impact on weight loss: Raising meat and fish on a grain-based diet rapidly increases their fat composition. But instead of the healthy fats you need, the result is a disproportionate amount of the fats that contribute to inflammation and cardiovascular disease.

Inflammation can lead to weight gain or an inability to lose weight. These animals are also lower in CLA (which fuels muscle development and fat loss) than their free range, grass fed, unfarmed counterparts

How to get rid of them: Change the way you shop for your meat and fish. Instead of searching for the occasional grass fed meat product or wild caught fish at your traditional supermarket, start shopping at local co-ops and farmers markets. Seek out local farmers who are raising chicken, beef, lamb, and pork using natural methods and buy from them.

Positive impact of elimination: Grass fed beef and high quality proteins such as pork and lamb that are properly pastured or raised in accordance with their natural needs and patterns are healthier, cleaner, free of antibiotics and hormones, lower in omega-6s, higher in omega-3s, and higher in conjugated linoleic acid (CLA); a compound that contributes to weight loss and muscle building.

Commercial Dairy Products

Milk is widely touted as a nutritional beverage, if not a requirement. However, the processes of pasteurization and homogenization, coupled with feedlot practices of corn-based diets, growth hormone injections, and antibiotics that later find their way into the finished product, make commercial dairy products anything but health-friendly.

Where you find them: Traditional, commercially produced milk and dairy products labelled pasteurized and homogenized, such as milk, cream, yogurt, cottage cheese, cream cheese, and sour cream. The word organic can be deceiving as many of these dairy products are still pasteurized and homogenized.

Why theyre harmful: Of special concern are the common practices within the mainstream dairy industry of feeding cows corn-based diets, giving growth hormones to dramatically increase milk production, and injecting harsh antibiotics to combat the rampant disease and infection that pervades overcrowded livestock conditions. These then pass into the milk found in traditional grocery store dairy aisles.

Consumption of these commercial dairy products has been linked to a wide range of conditions and ailments such as sinus problems, allergies, digestive distress, diabetes, rheumatoid arthritis, multiple sclerosis, and various cancers.

Negative impact on weight loss: The chemical-laden, pasteurized milk presents more of a risk than a benefit to the consumer. Pasteurization depletes milk of most of It's nutrients, thus making milk a source of empty calories. The process of pasteurization also changes the chemical composition of milk, making it harder for the human body to digest, and thus causing further strain on the digestive system.

How to get rid of them: Eliminating commercially produced and processed dairy products is easier than it may seem. Once you are able to shift your paradigm away from the idea of milk as a health food, it is as simple as changing the way you shop.

While many benefit from fully eliminating dairy products, another option is to switch to organic, raw dairy products.

Positive impact of elimination: Eliminating commercial dairy protects the body from a host of chemical additives and removes a source of empty calories. Many also experience improved skin conditions, diminished allergies, and relief from gas, bloating, and other digestive disorders.

Soy-Based Products

Though many jumped on the soy bandwagon in the search for better, healthier protein options, soy lacks the wholeness and nutrient richness of animal protein sources. Chemical processes used in commercial production of soy place it in the category of processed, nutrient-depleted foods to avoid for optimum health and weight loss.

Where you find them: Soy is widely used among the more upscale body of processed foods often labelled healthy or all-natural. Aside from soy in basic forms such as tofu, soymilk, and soy-based artificial meat products, soy is also found in protein powders, textured vegetable protein, and soy-protein energy bars.

Why theyre harmful: Unfermented soybeans contain toxins and anti-nutrients that can inhibit enzymes needed for digestion and absorption of nutrients. For example phytic acid, present in soy, inhibIt's the body's ability to absorb calcium, magnesium, copper, iron, and zinc.

Soy protein isolate is a filler substance of lowest quality and the chemical processes involved in It's production make it suspect from a safety perspective. Soy is also highly allergenic.

Negative impact on weight loss: When the body is depleted of essential minerals cravings result; often for unhealthy substitutes. Part of the problem with soy is that it replaces nutrient-rich food with a low-quality source of calories, which keeps the body from receiving the nutrients needed for proper functioning and metabolism. The hormones naturally occurring in soy also contribute to a sluggish metabolism and digestive system.

How to get rid of them: Don't use soy-based artificial meat products or tofu in place of quality, animal-based protein sources. Check labels on protein powders and energy bars for traces of soy protein isolate. If soymilk is a part of your diet, switch to raw cows milk or unsweetened nut milk, such as almond milk.

Positive impact of elimination: You may not be able to immediately perceive your body's increased ability to absorb nutrients or the proper regulation of hormones and metabolism, but these are the benefits of clearing your diet of soy-based foods.

Sports Drinks

Are sports drinks really necessary for hydration during sports and exercise? Or might water be sufficient to satisfy the body's needs? While sports drinks seem like the best way to fuel the exercise we need for weight loss, in reality they present one more hurdle to effectively reaching a healthy weight.

Where you find them: Though they come packaged under different brand names, these beverages are essentially the same. Gatorade and Powerade are most common, but many other beverage companies have developed sports lines as well.

Why theyre harmful: The marketing claims of sports drink companies are largely exaggerated. With the exception of elite athletes, few people exercise for such duration or in such extreme heat conditions as to necessitate such aggressive electrolyte and glucose replacement.

The citric acid present in these beverages weakens tooth enamel leading to decay and dental problems. These beverages also contain harmful chemical dyes and high fructose corn syrup. Sugar-free options are not beneficial as they contain harmful artificial sweeteners.

Negative impact on weight loss: Though generally thought to be a natural and necessary part of an active, healthy lifestyle, sports drinks provide little more than empty calories. The calorie-burning effects of exercise are cancelled in favour of an unnecessary beverage. These drinks also upset the body's natural processes of electrolyte replacement causing water retention and bloating,

How to get rid of them: Instead of reaching for the Gatorade, fill a bottle with natural, purified water for drinking during exercise. If you desire flavour, add a squeeze of lemon or lime. Iced herbal teas such as mint or hibiscus can also provide a healthy alternative and are as effective as water for the purpose of hydration.

Positive impact of elimination: Removing sports drinks removes unnecessary calories from your diet and helps to ensure that you are getting the quantity of pure water your body needs for hydration during physical activity.

Processed & Pre-packaged Foods

Though convenient and inexpensive, processed and pre-packaged foods introduce chemicals, toxins, and empty calories into the body which hamper weight loss and threaten overall good health.

Where you find them: There is no end to the creativity and scope of the offerings of the industrial, commercial food industry. Even the produce aisle now contains foods that have been processed or packaged for your convenience.

Packaged deli meats, boxed meals, canned soups, frozen dinners (even healthy varieties), low-calorie, lite, and diet products all fall under the processed, pre-packaged umbrella.

Why theyre harmful: These food products contain a long list of chemical dyes, flavour enhancers, preservatives, fillers and additives, sugars, and often trans fats. Your body was not designed to ingest these laboratory-created ingredients!

Negative impact on weight loss: Many of these foods also contain MSG; a known weight-loss inhibitor. Flavour enhancers and chemical sweeteners also tend to stimulate cravings and depress feelings of satiety, causing you to eat more.

How to get rid of them: Go through your pantry and

refrigerator and begin reading the labels on packages. Lots of ingredients you can't pronounce? Throw it away. When shopping, stick to the perimeter of the store, choosing fresh fruits and vegetables, natural meats and fish, eggs, and healthy grains. Buy organic whenever possible and seek out co-ops, natural food stores, and farmers markets.

Positive impact of elimination: Eating foods in their natural form ensures that you receive the full scope of nutrients and health benefits they have to offer as well as the natural fibre that assists weight loss. The result is a satisfied, healthy, energetic body. For many it also means the elimination of the physical and psychological side effects and allergic reactions caused by chemical food.

SUMMARY (Foods to Avoid):

- Products made with refined flour and corn cause an insulin response that prompts the body to store fat. For optimal weight loss, avoid cookies, pastas, and baked goods made with refined flours.

- Eliminate all products containing high fructose corn syrup. This product stimulates cravings, causes the body to store fat, and is a source of empty calories.

- Fake fats and hydrogenated vegetable and seed oils are harmful to the body and a major contributor to cardiovascular disease. Remove them from your kitchen and avoid fried foods when eating in restaurants.

- Artificial sweeteners are toxic to the body in all forms and their full danger is not completely known. Though non-sugar, they mimic sugar and fool the body into storing fat.

- Commercially raised meat and chicken and farm raised fish are low in nutrients and high in harmful fats, antibiotics, growth hormones; all of which contribute to inflammation and poor cardiovascular health.

- Commercially produced dairy products labelled pasteurized and homogenized are nutritionally depleted and rife with antibiotics, growth hormone, and the by-products of the cows GMO corn-based diet. These dairy products are chemically laden and a source of empty calories.

- Far from being a healthy protein option, soy products comprise a low-quality and even harmful food group that does not serve the body nutritionally.

- Don't confuse sports drinks with healthy beverage options. They are full of sugar and/or chemical additives, not to mention expensive and unnecessary.

- Clean your pantry and refrigerator of processed and pre-packaged foods to avoid harmful chemicals, low-quality ingredients, and empty calories.

THE FOODS TO EAT TO LOSE WEIGHT, LIVE LONGER & ENJOY A HEALTHY LIFESTYLE

Grass-Fed Raw Milk and Raw Dairy Products

Raw milk and raw dairy products come from cows that have been fed the grass-based diets they were designed to eat. The milk is free of harmful growth hormones and antibiotics and does not undergo the processes of pasteurization and homogenization.

Benefits for health and weight loss: Unlike traditional dairy products, which have been severely depleted of nutrients and can even cause weight gain, raw dairy products are nutrient rich and high in the proteins, enzymes, and naturally occurring vitamins and minerals that promote good health and weight loss.

Raw dairy products are also rich in saturated fat, which is hardly the diet danger it is reputed to be. Saturated fat from healthy cows promotes healthy cell repair, organ function, and feelings of satiety.

The conjugated linoleic acid (CLA) found in raw milk also aids the body's metabolic processes and helps to eliminate belly fat. CLA promotes immune function, muscle development, and overall good health.

Full of nutrients and free of hormones and antibiotics, raw milk and raw dairy products from grass-fed cows are a healthful part of an effective weight loss program.

Where to find it: Raw milk and dairy products are typically not found in commercial grocery stores. Instead, seek out co-ops and natural food stores in your area. Many farmers market vendors also sell raw milk or can provide a connection to a farmer in your area who does. Fine cheese shops frequently carry raw milk varieties.

High Quality Animal Proteins

When animals live in cleaner, healthier, more natural conditions and eat the diet that is right for them (instead of massive quanities of corn to fatten them up) they offer higher quality meat full of the nutrients, protein, and fat the body needs for proper health and weight loss. Seek out grass fed beef and bison, pork and lamb that has been farm raised with natural, organic feed, and wild caught fish.

Why is it better? When animals receive high quality feed and are raised outside of cramped pens, their bodies function properly and are less susceptible to stress and infection. While you pay a little more, the product more than delivers in terms of nutritional value and health safety.

Though corn and other low-quality grains fatten animals such as cows and fish quickly and cheaply, they also causes untold stress on their digestive systems, causing their bodies to mount an immune and hormone response.

Antibiotics are often required. Stress hormones like cortisol are then present in the finished product. Corn also causes rapid fat gain in the animal. While this is beneficial for the farmer, this fat is high in omega-6s.

Benefits for health and weight loss: High quality animal proteins that are raised naturally on their proper diet offer nutrients and proteins that your body can access easily. Naturally raised meats and fish are also high in Omega-3 fatty acids, which contribute to proper cell function and repair, disease prevention, decreased inflammation and insulin response, and a healthy metabolism.

The body requires a high quantity of protein for weight loss and satiation of hunger. When your protein is free of harmful chemicals and unheatlhy fats, you can eat the amount required to satisfy the needs of your body; the result is increased muscle and decreased body fat.

Proper protein consumption also helps to prevent diseases such as Type II diabetes, and improves metabolic function. If you are going to be consuming the high level of protein that you need for health and weight loss, you want to make sure that it is the best available.

Where to find it: Look carefully for beef and bison that have received a 100% grass based diet as some farmers and meat producers finish with corn but still label the beef grass fed. Make sure that the fish you buy is wild caught. Pork does not need to be grass fed, but ensure that the pork you purchased has received high quality organic feed.

Many co-ops and natural grocery stores carry these, but for the best value, find a farmer in your area and buy in bulk. If you are a hunter or have access to game meats, these are also an excellent protein option as they have lived in their natural environment, eaten their natural diet, and are free of hormones and antibiotics.

Free Range Chicken & Organic Free Range Eggs

Instead of being raised unable to move in a pen, free-range chickens are able to exercise and feed outside of a cage. Their feed is organic and does not contain GMO corn.

Benefits for health and weight loss: Animals living in environments that simulate their natural surroundings are contented and healthy and thus produce meats and products that are higher in nutrients and healthy fats.

They are less prone to illness and thus do not require antibiotics. As a result the food we get from these animals meets our nutritional needs, is satisfying, and tastes wonderful!

Free-range chickens and eggs provide proper omega-3/omega-6 ratios and are higher in nutrients than their commercial counterparts. Both are economical protein sources, versatile, and certainly an important part of a healthy diet and weight loss program.

Where to find them: Many traditional grocery stores are now beginning to carry organic, free-range eggs and chickens. They are commonly found at natural food stores and co-ops. You may also be able to purchase free-range chickens and eggs from a local farmer or farmers market.

Raw Nuts

Nuts are a fat and as shown in the previous section, certain fats are detrimental to health and weight loss efforts. But not all fats are created equal. Nuts provide essential vitamins and minerals and do not undergo the chemical processes associated with fake fats, hydrogenated oils, or trans fats.

Which nuts? All nuts have their own unique vitamin and mineral makeups but each provides a source of healthy fat that helps the body to feel satisfied and aids weight loss. Choose almonds, walnuts, Brazil nuts, pecans, pistachios, cashews, macadamia nuts, pine nuts, and hazelnuts.

Benefits for health and weight loss: The body definitely needs fats for proper brain function, cell repair, and to help the body feel satiated. Nuts are a healthy, natural source of the fats the body needs. They also provide sustained energy without an insulin response and help to diminish cravings.

Nuts are high in vitamins and minerals such as selenium, copper, manganese, zinc, magnesium, and vitamin E. The healthy fat in nuts helps lower the risk of cardiovascular disease and various cancers.

While overconsumption of fats can certainly contribute to weight gain, there is no need to fear fat. Nuts are a part of a balanced weight loss program and are a high quality food that meets a multitude of the body's needs. Good fats like nuts are important and far from actually making you fat, eaten in moderation they aid weight loss.

Where to find them: Look for raw nuts in all varieties as roasted nuts are often processed with harmful vegetable and seed oils. For highest quality nuts, buy them in the bulk section of your co-op or natural food store.

Berries

Berries are high in vitamins, antioxidants, and fibre. Low in carbohydrates, they provide a nutrient rich and delightfully sweet snack or addition to a meal.

Which berries? All berries including strawberries, blackberries, blueberries, raspberries, Goji berries, acai berries and even less common varieties such as loganberries, currants, and cranberries are high in nutritional benefits and a perfect part of a healthy weight loss program.

Benefits for health and weight loss: When your body receives the nutrients it needs, it is less likely to crave unhealthy foods or hold onto fat. Berries are rich in vitamins and minerals like vitamin C, folic acid, calcium, magnesium, and potassium.

Low in sugar and high in fibre, berries help guard against the blood sugar and insulin surges that cause the body to store fat. Consumption of berries has also been linked to improved vision, lowered risk of cancer, higher immunity, and protection of the skin.

Berries are an ideal way to satisfy cravings for sweet foods. Instead of a sugary dessert following a meal, enjoy a bowl of colourful, flavourful berries.

Where to find them: Berries can be found in any conventional grocery store, but it is important to purchase organic varieties as berries retain high levels of pesticides. Go out to a farm where you can pick your own or when in season, purchase from your local farmers market.

Fruits

In addition to berries, fruits of all varieties are an essential part of an effective weight loss program. Fruits are high in fibre, full of flavour, and packed with the vitamins and nutrients your body needs.

Which Fruits? While familiar fruits like apples, oranges, and bananas are excellent choices you can bring a little variety to your diet by experimenting with more exotic and tropical options. Many of these Fruits pack a powerful nutrient and antioxidant punch. Look for pineapple, papaya, mango, pomegranate, figs, kiwi, and apricots.

Benefits for health and weight loss: Fruits are naturally high in fibre, which aids weight loss by helping to remove toxins and other harmful substances from the body. Fibre helps you to feel satisfied longer after a meal and lowers insulin response. Diets rich in fibre also help to guard against cancers of the digestive system.

Fruit does contain natural sugar so it should be eaten in moderation, but on the whole, fruit is a perfect snack or a sweet addition to the end of the meal. As you develop a love for the rich and exotic flavours of fruits, cravings for fake sweeteners, processed sweets and desserts, and other unhealthy junk foods diminish.

Where to find them: You get the greatest nutritional benefits when you purchase organic produce in season.

Shop your local farmers market as the seasons permit. For exotic and tropical varieties, check ethnic marketsin your area; they often carry delicious fruits from Asia and Latin America.

Butter (from Grass Fed Cows)

Like other dairy products from grass-fed cows, this butter is higher in the nutrients and fats your body needs for proper functioning.

Why is it better? Butter contains milk solids and thus industrial feedlot butter carries the same risks and negative side effects of conventional milk and dairy products. When compared to margarine and other industrially produced and processed fats, butter is the far superior, weight loss-friendly, natural option.

Butter also tastes better and thus helps you to feel satisfied after meals. Remember, not all things that taste good are bad for you! Which would you prefer: rich, natural butter or chemical margarine?

Benefits for health and weight loss: In addition to simply tasting better and providing a higher quality source of fat, butter contains essential fatty acids, is rich in vitamins such as A, K, and D, and also contains conjugated linoleic acid (CLA) which helps to reduce body fat, build muscle, and stimulate metabolic health.

Where to find it: Always purchase organic grass-fed butter as pesticides and chemicals are easily stored in fat. High quality organic butters can be found at your local co-op or natural foods store and are becoming increasingly common in conventional supermarkets as well.

Vegetables

Vegetables need little introduction. We have long been told of their benefits though rarely eat enough of them. Did you know vegetables are an essential part of your weight reduction plan?

Which vegetables? While all vegetables contribute to a healthy diet and weight loss program, some are higher in nutritional value than others. Dark leafy greens such as kale, collards, chard, and spinach top the list of vegetables that belong in any diet.

It is also good to eat from a wide range of colours and textures. Not only does this pattern of eating help you to experience a wide variety of vitamins, phenols, and polyphenols (from vegetable pigments), it also spices uyour diet and keeps you feeling satisfied.

Benefits for health and weight loss: Listing the benefits of the wide world of edible plant foods would take volumes. Vegetables are rich in vitamins and minerals and provide the essential elements for proper health and physical functioning. And as has been demonstrated, when the body receives both the macro- and micronutrients it requires, inflammation and insulin response decrease, and the body is free to seek a healthy weight.

High fibre vegetables are also our best defence against cancer. Research has yet to fully elucidate the cancer and disease-fighting properties of the vegetables available to us. Eat as many as you can!

Vegetables are loaded with nutrients are thus a good snack when the craving for something crunchy hits. While celery sticks may not initially be as appealing as a stack of cookies, with time your body will grow to crave these natural delights.

Where to find them: Again, organic is best and local is even better. Shop farmers markets and local co-ops to obtain produce grown in your area.

Natural Oils

The body can't function without fat and those looking to lose weight need not fear it. Unlike factory-produced oils, vegetable and seed oils, fake fats, margarine, and trans fats, natural fats enhance the body's natural processes without causing a harmful inflammatory response.

Which oils? Choose extra virgin olive oil for flavouring foods and for making dressings and sauces. Coconut oil, which is perfectly stable at high temperatures, is best for sauting, stir-frying, and other cooking done over high heat.

Benefits for health and weight loss: Mediterranean countries have been using olive oil for centuries and not coincidentally have a far lower risk of cancer, cardiovascular disease, and obesity than nations dependent on chemical and trans fats.

Coconut oil is an amazing product and a perfect cooking option for those looking to lose weight. Coconut oil aids weight loss efforts by providing sustained energy, promoting healthy thyroid function, and helping the body to burn fat.

Where to find them: Coconut oil is now available at many grocery stores. Olive oil, though widely available, requires careful label reading. Look for organic, high-quality extra virgin olive oil from small producers.

Whole Grains and Complex Carbohydrates

Whole, natural, unprocessed grains, eaten in moderation can be a part of a healthy weight loss program. Many are high in protein and fibre and provide bulk to the diet.

Which grains? Not all grains are created equal. Though refined white flour technically comes from a grain, it is processed to the point that it is not only nutritionally deficient, but even harmful to the body. Healthy grains and carbohydrates include whole grain brown rice, quinoa, amaranth, oats, sweet potatoes, and all varieties of starchy beans and lentils.

Benefits for health and weight loss: Unlike their over-processed counterparts, natural grains, beans, and sweet potatoes, cause a much subtler insulin response in the body due to their low glycemic index and high levels of fibre.

Healthy grains help provide bulk in the diet and are a readily available source of energy for physical activity. Sweet potatoes are especially beneficial for post-workout recovery, and grains like bulgur and quinoa make a great addition to salads or a healthier alternative to white rice and pasta.

Where to find them: Many grocery stores have begun to carry a wider variety of grains and beans. Co-ops and natural food stores often carry these items in bulk, allowing you to try small quantities to discover new favourites.

Natural Sweeteners

Though natural sweeteners are still sugars and should only be consumed in moderate to small amounts, they have a weight loss edge over traditional refined white sugar, high fructose corn syrup, and artificial sweeteners.

Which sweeteners? For cooking and baking, or for sweetening food and drinks, natural sweeteners such as raw organic honey, natural maple syrup, and blackstrap molasses are the best choices. Stevia, a plant based natural sweetener is calorie free and potently sweet.

Benefits for health and weight loss: Natural sweeteners (with the exception of stevia) still contain calories and can trigger cravings for sweet foods. Thus these sweeteners should only be consumed only occasionally for best weight loss results.

Honey has long been praised for it's many health benefits. Beyond it's unique taste and liquid sweetness, honey can actually help your body process glucose, is high in various vitamins, and contains antioxidants and antibacterial properties as well.

Real maple syrup and blackstrap molasses also contain minerals and antioxidants. Stevia, which has been popular in Latin America for many years, is an all-natural sweetener, safe to use, and completely calorie free.

Where to find them: Natural, organic honeys and

syrups as well as stevia can be found at specialty stores or co-ops or, in the case of honey and maple syrup, purchased from the producer directly.

Dark Chocolate

Low in sugar and highly satisfying, dark chocolate is the perfect sweet treat. It's intense flavour helps to guard against over-indulgence. It's full of powerful antioxidants as well; you can't say that about those store-bought baked goods!

Which type of chocolate? The better the grade and quality the chocolate, the greater the benefits. Chocolate labels will contain a percentage number that indicates the quantity of pure cocoa. The higher this number, the lower the percentage of sugar and cocoa butter. Look for 70% cocoa or higher.

Benefits for health and weight loss: High in flavonoids, dark chocolate boasts superior antioxidant properties. Dark chocolate also promotes heart health, brain functioning, and even emotional stability

Dark chocolate is a natural mood-enhancer and relaxer; even in small quantities. Eating a square or two helps you to feel satisfied and diminishes the feelings of deprivation associated with most diets.

Where to find it: High quality dark chocolate can be purchased from upscale candy stores and is also increasingly available in co-ops and even conventional grocery stores. Look for a pure cocoa level of 70% or higher.

Water

Though it seems obvious, water deserves a place in any weight loss regimen. Simple as it is, the benefits of proper water intake cannot be overstated.

Which water? You need not drink fancy bottled varieties in order to reap the benefits of water, but a home purifier may help to remove unwanted minerals from your water and improve it's flavour. Some prefer mineral water or something with a little fizz. As long as you are drinking water (at least 8 glasses a day), the type of water is simply a matter of preference.

Benefits for health and weight loss: Water hydrates the body from the inside out allowing it to function properly. Water cleanses the body of toxins that can inhibit weight loss, increases energy, and keeps the body in overall good health.

Water also helps with weight loss efforts by helping to regulate hunger. Many times the sensation of hunger between meals is actually thirst. Before reaching for a snack, drink a large glass of water and see if it does the trick.

Essential for exercising and athletic activity, water helps improve endurance and stamina, keeping the body well hydrated and replacing fluids lost through sweat.

Where to find your water: If the flavour of your tap

water deters you from drinking it, consider purchasing a filter. Keep a water bottle on you at all times to remind you to continue drinking throughout the day; even when you arent exercising. Specialty mineral waters, which are a nice treat, can be purchased at grocery stores or natural food stores

SUMMARY (Foods to Eat):

- Raw milk is free of the chemicals, antibiotics, and growth hormones that plague conventional dairy products. Far from being harmful or nutritionally devoid as a result of the pasteurization process, raw milk is rich in healthy fats and nutrients that promote weight loss.

- Grass fed beef, bison, and lamb, naturally raised pork and wild caught fish are the highest quality source of protein and rich in fats associated with good cardiovascular health. These animals are also free of the harmful hormones, antibiotics, and diseases that plague feedlot animals.

- Organic, free range chicken and eggs provide a healthier source of protein than chickens raised in overpopulated cages. Both free-range poultry and eggs are richer in nutrients and omega-3 fatty acids.

- Like other good fats, nuts promote feelings of satiety, provide sustained energy, and are a source of vital minerals.

- Berries are high in vitamins, antioxidants, and fibre, but low in calories making them a perfect sweet treat and a healthy addition to meals.

- Fruits of all varieties provide health benefits and a

lower calorie option for healthy snacks. Eat a wide variety of Fruits for greatest benefit.

- Unlike it's commercially produced, feedlot counterpart, grass-fed butter is rich in the fats that actually promote fat loss.

- Vegetables in all forms satisfy the body's myriad of nutritional needs. High in fibre and low in calories, vegetables, especially dark, leafy varieties, should be a daily addition to the diet.

- Natural oils such as olive oil and coconut oil are superior to commercially produced vegetable and seed oils and fake fats. They aid the body's natural processes, promote proper metabolic function, and do not cause an inflammatory response.

- Whole, unprocessed grains and sweet potatoes are a healthy source of carbohydrates and provide bulk to the diet.

- Instead of refined sugars, high fructose corn syrup, or other artificial sweeteners, choose honey, maple syrup, blackstrap molasses, or stevia to lightly sweeten foods.

- Dark chocolate, rich in antioxidants, provides a healthier option for a sweet treat. It also brightens your mood and promotes relaxation.

- Water is essential not only for hydration during

exercise but for daily physical functioning. It also supresses appetite. Make sure to drink at least 8 glasses per day.

THE 'LITTLE-KNOWN' BUT MOST POWERFUL FAT LOSS SECRET EVER DEVELOPED

One of the most closely held secrets of the fitness and modelling industry is ... "Carb Cycling".

Probably the most powerful fat loss secret on the planet, carb cycling can help you lose weight quickly, without stalling your metabolism, and without losing muscle.

Consuming less calories than your body burns off everyday, will enable you to lose weight, but as we discussed earlier in this report, consuming far less calories over an extended period of time will trigger your body's starvation response and bring your metabolism to a screeching halt.

Making permanent weight loss a nightmare!

However, by following carb cycling, your body reaps the benefits of lower calories, without the negative effects on your metabolism.

In a nutshell, you will be eating a low carbohydrate diet 3 days per week, followed by 1 or 2 days on a higher carb diet.

So in effect, you are eating less calories for 3 days, but the important point is, you are eating less carb calories.

Here's how it works:

By eating less carb calories for 3 days, your insulin response is kept very low and before your body has a chance to trigger the starvation response and slow down its natural ability to burn fat, you load up on carbs on day 4.

Then the cycle continues.

Bodybuilders, use this exact strategy to get ripped and defined muscles, and the only way to do that is by having less than 8% fat on their body, so it's deadly effective.

And it's not nearly as difficult as you'd believe.

To make it simple, as you already know, I believe calorie counting is a waste of time and energy and just leads to confusion for most people.

So here's what you should do.

3 days per week, I want you to have a small serving of carbohydrates OR fruit with your breakfast and that's it.

The rest of the day on those 3 days you will be consuming animal protein, healthy fats, and preferably leafy green vegetables. But, no sandwiches for lunch and pasta or potatoes are out for dinner. Just healthy proteins, fats and vegetables from our approved categories in the last chapter.

On day 4, you can up your carbs, but remember to choose foods from our approved categories.

So you will still be eating a balanced diet of proteins, fats and vegetables but you can have a serving of carbohydrates with as many meals as you want. This will replenish the glucagon levels in your body, raise your insulin, satisfy you no end, and boost your metabolism on the back of the lower carb days.

There are no hard and fast rules. But never have more than 2 high days in a row and never have more than 3 low days in a row.

This strategy combined with the food choices we discussed in the last chapters, is an extremely powerful combination which will see you shedding pounds in no time.

Conclusion: The New, Leaner, Healthier You Starts Right Now

Obesity is more prevalent today that is was just a few short years ago, and that is because of the conflicting advice, and ABUNDANCE of diet reports and plans that do nothing but lose you weight temporarily, aside from that like I mentioned before, most diets will have you restricting calories, which slows down your metabolism and prevents you from getting adequate nutrition.

The truly great thing about eating a healthy diet, rich in nutrients, like nature intended … is that you will NOT experience DRASTIC hunger pangs, you'll feel satisfied, will NOT crave junk food, you'll be happier AND lighter too.

Just give it 14 days … and remember;

- Don't believe conventional wisdom, the food industry or the government. The food pyramid will do nothing but make you fat and nutrient deprived.

- Consuming genetically modified, highly processed and refined carbohydrate rich foods will make you fat!

- The fewer carbs and empty calories you eat, the leaner you'll be.

- The carbs to avoid are; (sugars, starches, refined flour, pasta and bread unless fortified), not leafy green vegetables and salads.

- You can eat all you want of animal protein (yes, even red meat) on a natural diet and healthy fats.

- Eat when you are hungry and until full. If you are not eating empty calories, you wont get fat or any fatter.

- Cutting back calories in the diet to lose weight wont work if you do not cut back on GM, processed and refined carbs because you'll be constantly hungry, nutrient deprived, your metabolism will stall and insulin levels will rise.

- Avoid trans-fat at all costs.

Like this report?

Thanks for purchaing and reading this report. I'm positive if you just follow this plan, you will reach your weight loss goals a lot easier and quicker than you realize. However, could you spare one minute and do me a quick favour though?

If you found this report useful, would you leave me a positive review on Amazon?

I love getting feedback and knowing I'm helping people makes a real difference to me. I read all my reviews and would really appreciate your thoughts. A 5 star review on Amazon is like giving me a tip for $20.

... And I would very, very much appreciate the gesture.

To leave a review, please visit:

http://amzn.to/13yawnk

Thanks again and I wish you the best of luck.

Your trusted friend,

Jennifer James

DISCLAIMER AND/OR LEGAL NOTICES: Every effort has been made to accurately represent this report and it's potential. Results vary with every individual, and your results may or may not be different from those depicted. No promises, guarantees or warranties, whether stated or implied, have been made that you will produce any specific result from this report. Your efforts are individual and unique, and may vary from those shown. Your success depends on your efforts, background and motivation.

The material in this publication is provided for educational and informational purposes only and is not intended as medical advice. The information contained in this report should not be used to diagnose or treat any illness, metabolic disorder, disease or health problem. Always consult your physician or health care provider before beginning any nutrition or exercise program. Use of the programs, advice, and information contained in this report is at the sole choice and risk of the reader.